This report contains the collective views of an international group of experts and does not necessarily represent the decisions or the stated policy of the United Nations Environment Programme, the International Labour Organisation, or the World Healt Organization.

**Environmental Health Criteria 170**

# ASSESSING HUMAN HEALTH RISKS OF CHEMICALS: DERIVATION OF GUIDANCE VALUES FOR HEALTH-BASED EXPOSURE LIMITS

Published under the joint sponsorship of
the United Nations Environment Programme,
the International Labour Organisation,
and the World Health Organization

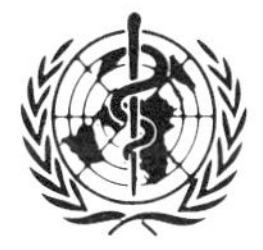

World Health Organization
Geneva, 1994

The **International Programme on Chemical Safety (IPCS)** is a joint venture of the United Nations Environment Programme, the International Labour Organisation, and the World Health Organization. The main objective of the IPCS is to carry out and disseminate evaluations of the effects of chemicals on human health and the quality of the environment. Supporting activities include the development of epidemiological, experimental laboratory, and risk-assessment methods that could produce internationally comparable results, and the development of manpower in the field of toxicology. Other activities carried out by the IPCS include the development of know-how for coping with chemical accidents, coordination of laboratory testing and epidemiological studies, and promotion of research on the mechanisms of the biological action of chemicals.

WHO Library Cataloguing in Publication Data

Assessing human health risks of chemicals : derivation of guidance values for health-based exposure limits.

(Environmental health criteria ; 170)

1.Hazardous substances - toxicity 2.Environmental exposure 3.Guidelines I.Series

ISBN 92 4 157170 5 (NLM Classification: WA 465)
ISSN 0250-863X



PRINTED IN FINLAND
94/10274 – VAMMALA – 5500

## CONTENTS

ENVIRONMENTAL HEALTH CRITERIA FOR GUIDANCE VALUES FOR HUMAN EXPOSURE LIMITS

## WHO TASK GROUP ON ENVIRONMENTAL HEALTH CRITERIA FOR GUIDANCE VALUES FOR HUMAN EXPOSURE LIMITS

*Members*

Dr D. Anderson[c], British Industrial and Biological Research Association (BIBRA), Carshalton, Surrey, United Kingdom

Professor B. Baranski[b], Nofer's Institute of Occupational Medicine, Lodz, Poland

Dr V. Benes[b], Toxicology and Reference Laboratory, Institute of Hygiene and Epidemiology, Prague, Czech Republic

Dr T. DeRosa[a], Division of Toxicology, Agency for Toxic Substances and Disease Registry, Atlanta, Georgia, USA

Dr M. Dourson[a, b, c ||], Systemic Toxicants Assessment Branch, Environmental Criteria and Assessments Office, Office of Research and Development, US Environmental Protection Agency, Cincinnati, Ohio, USA

Dr J. Duffus[c], Department of Biological Sciences, The Edinburgh Centre for Toxicology, Herriot-Watt University, Edinburgh, United Kingdom

Dr E. Dybing[a /], Department of Environmental Medicine, National Institute of Public Health, Oslo, Norway

Dr R.J. Fielder[c], Department of Health, Elephant and Castle, London, United Kingdom

Dr T. Harvey[b, c], Environmental Criteria and Assessment Office, US Environmental Protection Agency, Cincinnati, Ohio, USA

Dr R. Hasegawa[c], Division of Toxicology Safety, National Institute of Health Sciences, Setagaya-ku, Tokyo, Japan

Dr E. Kamata[a], National Institute of Health Sciences, Setagaya-ku, Tokyo, Japan

Dr A.G.A.C. Knaap[a, b, c], Toxicology Advisory Centre, National Institute of Public Health and Environmental Protection, Bilthoven, The Netherlands

Dr M.E. Meek[a II, b II, c I], Environmental Health Directorate, Health Protection Branch, Health and Welfare, Ottawa, Ontario, Canada

Dr E. Poulsen[b], Humlebaek, Denmark

Dr A.G. Renwick[a II, b II, c II], Clinical Pharmacology Group, University of Southampton, Medical and Biological Sciences Building, Southampton, United Kingdom

Dr A.E. Robinson[a], Toronto, Ontario, Canada

Professor J.A. Sokal[b], Institute of Occupational Medicine and Environmental Health, Sosnowiec, Poland

Dr R. Türck[a, b I, c], Federal Ministry of Environment, Nature Conservation and Nuclear Safety, Bonn, Germany

Professor F. Valic[b, c], Department of Occupational Health, Andrija Štampar School of Public Health, Zagreb University, Zagreb, Croatia

Dr G.A. Zapponi[b], Laboratory of Environmental Health, Istituto Superiore di Sanità, Rome, Italy

*Representatives of other Organizations*

Mr S. Arai[a, b], Organisation for Economic Co-operation and Development, Paris, France

Dr P. Boffetta[a], International Agency for Research on Cancer, Lyon, France

Dr J. Furlong[b], Directorate-General XI A.2, Environment, Nuclear Safety and Civil Protection, Commission of the European Communities, Brussels, Belgium

Mr S. Machida[a], Occupational Safety and Health Branch, Working Conditions and Environment Department, International Labour Office, Geneva, Switzerland

Dr H. Moller[c], International Agency for Research on Cancer, Lyon, France

Dr V. Morgenroth[c], Organisation for Economic Co-operation and Development, Paris, France

Ms F. Ouane[a], International Register of Potentially Toxic Chemicals, United Nations Environment Programme, Geneva, Switzerland

Ms A. Sunden[a], International Register of Potentially Toxic Chemicals, United Nations Environment Programme, Geneva, Switzerland

*Observers*

Dr G.P. Daston[c], Procter & Gamble, Miami Valley Laboratories, Cincinnati, Ohio, USA

Dr He Fengsheng[c], Division of Health Protection and Promotion, World Health Organization, Geneva, Switzerland

Dr C. Lally[c], Procter & Gamble, European Technical Centre, Stombeek-Bever, Belgium

Dr D. Mage[a, c], Division of Environment Health, Prevention of Environmental Pollution, World Health Organization, Geneva, Switzerland

Dr M.I. Mikheev[a], Office of Occupational Health, World Health Organization, Geneva, Switzerland

Professor G. Di Renzo[c], Department of Human Communication Science, Faculty of Medicine, Frederico II University, Naples, Italy

Dr J.A. Stober[a], Division of Environment Health, World Health Organization, Geneva, Switzerland

Dr G. Würtzen[b, c], Coca-Cola International, Glostrup Centre, Glostrup, Denmark

*Secretariat*

Dr G. Becking[a, c], International Programme on Chemical Safety, Interregional Research Unit, World Health Organization, Research Triangle Park, North Carolina, USA

Dr H. Galal-Gorchev[a], International Programme on Chemical Safety, World Health Organization, Geneva, Switzerland

Dr J. Herrman[a], International Programme on Chemical Safety, World Health Organization, Geneva, Switzerland

Dr D. Kello[b], World Health Organization, Regional Office for Europe, Copenhagen, Denmark

Mr D. Schutz[a], International Programme on Chemical Safety, World Health Organization, Geneva, Switzerland

Dr E. Smith[a, b, c], International Programme on Chemical Safety, World Health Organization, Geneva, Switzerland

Mr K. Tanaka[a], International Programme on Chemical Safety, World Health Organization, Geneva, Switzerland

Dr M. Younes[b, c], European Centre for Environment and Health, World Health Organization, Bilthoven, The Netherlands

---

[a] Participated in IPCS Discussions on Methodology for Establishing Guidance Values (GV) for Various Exposure Situations, Geneva, Switzerland, 14-17 January 1992

[b] Participated in WHO EURO/IPCS Consultation on Guiding Principles and Methodology for Quantitative Risk Assessment in Setting Exposure Limits, Langen, Germany, 19-22 January 1993

[c] Participated in WHO Task Group Meeting on Risk Assessment Methodology (Guidance Values), Geneva, Switzerland, 14-18 June 1993

[i] Chairman of meeting

[ii] Joint Rapporteur

## NOTE TO READERS OF THE CRITERIA MONOGRAPHS

Every effort has been made to present information in the criteria monographs as accurately as possible without unduly delaying their publication. In the interest of all users of the Environmental Health Criteria monographs, readers are kindly requested to communicate any errors that may have occurred to the Director of the International Programme on Chemical Safety, World Health Organization, Geneva, Switzerland, in order that they may be included in corrigenda.

* * *

A detailed data profile and a legal file can be obtained from the International Register of Potentially Toxic Chemicals, Case postale 356, 1219 Châtelaine, Geneva, Switzerland (Telephone No. 9799111).

* * *

This publication was made possible by grant number 5 U01 ES02617-15 from the National Institute of Environmental Health Sciences, National Institutes of Health, USA, and by financial support from the European Commission.

## ENVIRONMENTAL HEALTH CRITERIA FOR GUIDANCE VALUES FOR HUMAN EXPOSURE LIMITS

This Environmental Health Criteria monograph was developed in the course of three meetings, i) a Discussion Group, World Health Organization, Geneva, Switzerland, 14-17 January 1992, opened by Dr E. Smith, IPCS, ii) a Consultation, Langen, Germany, 19-22 January 1993, opened by Dr D. Kello, World Health Organization, Regional Office for Europe, and iii) the final Task Group, World Health Organization, Geneva, 14-18 June 1993, opened by Dr E. Smith, IPCS.

Dr E. Smith and Dr P.G. Jenkins, both members of the IPCS Central Unit, were responsible for the overall scientific content and technical editing, respectively.

The WHO Regional Office for Europe collaborated with the International Programme on Chemical Safety in the development of the Guidance Value concept.

The German Federal Ministry for the Environment, Nature Conservation and Nuclear Safety provided funding support for the Consultation in Langen, Germany.

The efforts of all who helped in the preparation and finalization of the monograph are gratefully acknowledged.

# ABBREVIATIONS

| | |
|---|---|
| ADI | acceptable daily intake |
| AUC | area under the curve |
| EPI | exposure/potency index |
| LO(A)EL | lowest-observed-(adverse)-effect level |
| NO(A)EL | no-observed-(adverse)-effect level |
| SAR | structure-activity relationship |
| TI | tolerable intake |
| UF | uncertainty factor |

# SUMMARY

Guidance values for exposure to chemicals in environmental media should be developed in IPCS Environmental Health Criteria (EHC) monographs and can be modified by national and local authorities in their development of limits and standards for environmental media. For any chemical, the steps involved are:

1. Evaluate and summarize the information on toxicity in animals and humans and exposure in humans which is most relevant to derivation of guidance values. The most appropriate format for presentation of the data relevant to derivation of guidance values is a written narrative summarizing the critical data complemented by graphical presentation.

2. Such data can be used to derive a Tolerable Intake (TI) for various routes of exposure for effects considered to have a threshold. This will involve application of uncertainty factors, generally to the no-observed-adverse-effect level (NOAEL) for critical effects in the most relevant study. For non-threshold effects, the dose-response relationship will be characterized to the extent possible.

3. Estimate the proportion of total intake that originates from various media (e.g., indoor and ambient air, food and water), based on exposure estimates for a consistent set of assumed volumes of intake (using the International Commission on Radiological Protection (ICRP) reference man) and representative concentrations in the general environment, for a given situation. In the absence of adequate data on concentrations in various media, mathematical models may be used to estimate the distribution through the various media.

4. Allocate a proportion of the TI to various media of exposure (based on the exposure estimate described in step 3 above) to determine the intake or exposure in each medium.

5. Develop guidance values from intakes assigned to each medium, taking into account (if necessary) body weight, volume of intake and absorption efficiency (the *relative* absorption efficiency in situations where the guidance value is derived on the basis of a TI by another route of exposure). In EHC monographs, development of guidance values would be undertaken for a clearly defined exposure scenario, based on the data for ICRP reference

man, and not necessarily representative of national or local exposure conditions. Guidance values would commonly be derived for a representative general population with representative exposure conditions. The guidance values should be adapted at national and local levels as appropriate for local circumstances.

6. The basis for the derivation of both the TI and the guidance values should be described clearly in EHC monographs (see level of detail in examples in Appendix 1).

activity and considered to be critical to the derivation of sound guidance values in EHCs.

Many toxicological studies are directed mainly to hazard identification. The available data may not always contain sufficient information on the dose-response relationship for risk assessment and for the derivation of TIs for guidance values. Reports and publications in which no-observed-effect level (NOEL) or NOAEL values are presented should include sufficient information on all possible effects investigated and those observed or not observed to allow an assessment of the validity of the derived values.

## 1.4 Clarity and transparency of presentations

Data on the dose-response relationship for the critical effect which served as the basis for the derivation of the guidance values (GVs) should be characterized in EHC monographs to the extent possible (including graphical presentation, similar to that illustrated in Appendix 3 for benchmark doses). It is recognized that in many cases, the data base will be insufficient for provision of such information and that it may only be possible to develop single guidance values in individual media with little additional risk characterization. Similarly, the basis for the uncertainty factors by which the NOAEL or lowest-observable-adverse-effect level (LOAEL) have been divided to obtain the TI should be clearly specified. The conversion of the TI into media-specific GVs should be presented in sufficient detail to allow the values to be adapted to national or local circumstances (see examples in Appendix 1 for relevant level of detail).

# 2. GUIDANCE VALUES

## 2.1 General considerations

A consistent methodology should be used in the derivation of quantitative guidance values for human exposures to chemical substances present in food, drinking-water, air and other media by *ad hoc* IPCS Task Groups (of varying membership) reviewing and evaluating data and finalizing EHC monographs on various chemicals. This approach embodies the concept that, to the extent possible, guidance values for the protection of human health should reflect consideration of total exposure to the substance whether present in air, water, soil, food or other media. Guidance values should be derived for a clearly defined exposure scenario, based on the data for the ICRP reference man (Appendix 4), and therefore might not represent national or local circumstances.

### *2.1.1 Precision of a guidance value*

The precision of the guidance values is dependent upon the validity and reliability of the available data. Frequently, there are sources of uncertainty in the derivation of TIs (see section 4.8) and in their allocation as a basis for GVs, so that the resulting values represent a best estimate based on the available data at the time. A description of the derivation of guidance value should clearly indicate the nature and sources of uncertainty and the manner in which they have been taken into account in the derivation. The numerical value of GVs should reflect the precision present in their derivation; usually GVs should be given to only one significant figure.

## 2.2 Derivation of guidance values

Establishing TIs is central to the determination of guidance values. A TI is defined as:-

> an estimate of the intake of a substance over a lifetime that is considered to be without appreciable health risk. It may have different units depending upon the route of administration upon which it is based and is generally expressed on a daily or weekly basis. Though not strictly an "intake", TIs for inhalation are generally expressed as airborne concentrations (i.e. $\mu$g or mg per $m^3$). The TI is similar in definition and intent to terms such as reference dose (RfD) (Barnes &

Dourson, 1988), reference concentration (RfC) (Jarabek et al., 1990) and acceptable daily intake (ADI).

This monograph addresses two areas that are critical in the methodology for the derivation of guidance values for human exposures to chemical substances in the environment:

- *Development of a tolerable intake on the basis of interpretation of the available data on toxicity.* For practical purposes, toxic effects are considered to be of two types, threshold and non-threshold. For substances where the critical effect is considered to have a threshold (including non-genotoxic carcinogenesis for which there is adequate mechanistic data), a TI is developed usually on the basis of a NOAEL. Development of guidance values in EHC monographs for non-threshold effects (e.g., genotoxic carcinogenesis and germ cell mutations) is discussed in section 3.1.1.

- *Allocation of the proportions of the tolerable intake to various media.* Depending on available information, the development of guidance values for compounds present in more than one environmental medium will require the allocation of proportions of the TI to various media (for example, air, food and water). For the derivation of guidance values, the allocation will be based on information on relative exposure via different routes.

## 2.3 Interpretation and use of guidance values

Media exposure allocations of TIs for the derivation of guidance values in EHC monographs are based on relative exposure by different routes for a given scenario. Though this is suggested as a practical approach, the use of allocations based on exposure in different media does not preclude the development of more stringent limits. It is also important to recognize that the proportions of total intake from various media may vary, based on circumstances. Site- or context-specific guidance values better suited to local circumstances and conditions could be developed from TIs presented in the EHC in situations where relevant data on exposure are available, and particularly where there are other significant sources of exposure to a chemical substance (e.g., in the vicinity of a waste site). Regulatory authorities may also take other factors into account, such as cost, ease and effectiveness of control, to develop risk management strategies appropriate for local circumstances, although the ultimate objective of control should be reduction of exposure from all sources to less than the TIs. In addition, where data on organoleptic thresholds are included in EHC monographs, these can also be considered by relevant authorities in the development of limits.

The basis for derivation of guidance values in EHC monographs must be clearly specified in sufficient detail to enable, where appropriate, step-by-step development of exposure limits for national or local conditions by appropriate regulatory or other authorities (Appendix 1).

## 2.4 Terminology

**Adverse effect:** change in morphology, physiology, growth, development or life span of an organism which results in impairment of functional capacity or impairment of capacity to compensate for additional stress or increase in susceptibility to the harmful effects of other environmental influences. Decisions on whether or not any effect is adverse require expert judgement.

**Critical effect(s):** the adverse effect(s) judged to be most appropriate for determining the TI.

**No-observed-adverse-effect level (NOAEL):** greatest concentration or amount of a substance, found by experiment or observation, which causes no detectable adverse alteration of morphology, functional capacity, growth, development or life span of the target organism under defined conditions of exposure. Alterations of morphology, functional capacity, growth, development or life span of the target may be detected which are judged not to be adverse.

**No-observed-effect level (NOEL):** greatest concentration or amount of a substance, found by experiment or observation, that causes no alterations of morphology, functional capacity, growth, development or life span of target organisms distinguishable from those observed in normal (control) organisms of the same species and strain under the same defined conditions of exposure.

**Lowest-observed-adverse-effect level (LOAEL):** lowest concentration or amount of a substance, found by experiment or observation, which causes an adverse alteration of morphology, functional capacity, growth, development or life span of the target organism distinguishable from normal (control) organisms of the same species and strain under the same defined conditions of exposure.

**Benchmark dose:** the lower confidence limit of the dose calculated to be associated with a given incidence (e.g., 5 or 10% incidence) of effect estimated from all toxicity data on that effect within that study (Crump, 1984).

**Uncertainty factor (UF):** a product of several single factors by which the NOAEL or LOAEL of the critical effect is divided to derive a TI. These factors account for adequacy of the pivotal study, interspecies extrapolation, inter-individual variability in humans, adequacy of the overall data base, and nature of toxicity. The term uncertainty factor was considered to be a more appropriate expression than safety factor since it avoids the notion of absolute safety and because the size of this factor is proportional to the magnitude of uncertainty rather than safety. The choice of UF should be based on the available scientific evidence.

**Toxicodynamics:** the process of interaction of chemical substances with target sites and the subsequent reactions leading to adverse effects.

**Toxicokinetics:** the process of the uptake of potentially toxic substances by the body, the biotransformation they undergo, the distribution of the substances and their metabolites in the tissues, and the elimination of the substances and their metabolites from the body. Both the amounts and the concentrations of the substances and their metabolites are studied. The term has essentially the same meaning as pharmacokinetics, but the latter term should be restricted to the study of pharmaceutical substances.

**Tolerable intake (TI):** an estimate of the intake of a substance which can occur over a lifetime without appreciable health risk. It may have different units depending upon the route of administration. Though not strictly an "intake", TIs for inhalation are generally expressed as airborne concentrations (i.e., $\mu$g or mg per $m^3$).

**Default value:** pragmatic, fixed or standard value used in the absence of relevant data.

**Guidance values (GVs):** values, such as concentrations in air or water, which are derived after appropriate allocation of the TI among the different possible media of exposure. Combined exposures from all media at the guidance values over a lifetime would be expected to be without appreciable health risk. The aim of the guidance value is to provide quantitative information from risk assessment for risk managers to enable them to make decisions concerning the protection of human health.

# 3. APPLICATION OF THE TOXICITY DATA BASE TO DETERMINE TOLERABLE INTAKES

## 3.1 Approaches to risk assessment

A review of the data base on a chemical should be undertaken to determine the critical effect(s), which can be considered to be of two types: those considered to have a threshold and those for which there is considered to be some risk at any level (non-threshold: genotoxic carcinogens and germ cell mutagens). Data available for risk assessments include studies in humans and animals, structure-activity relationships (SAR) and *in vitro* investigations. Risk assessments should be based on all available data at the time of review, but it is appreciated that recognition of additional hazards or risk may emerge which will require subsequent re-evaluation. Wherever possible, appropriate human data should be used as the basis for the risk assessment.

For threshold effects, where data in humans are used as the basis for development of TIs, uncertainty factors should be applied to observed effect levels to allow for the magnitude of any effect seen in the exposed group and their sensitivity compared with the general population or target group. The incidence of effects detected in humans *in vivo* will be the result of inter-individual differences in both toxicokinetic and toxicodynamic aspects. The extent of any possible human variability not present within the exposed population groups should be considered in the development of uncertainty factors.

Information on the NOAEL (or LOAEL) by different routes is sometimes available. In cases where information exists on only one route, e.g., inhalation, the bioequivalence for exposure from other routes should be estimated if suitable information and models are available. The aim of the risk assessment is to estimate an overall tolerable intake derived from data on toxicity using appropriate routes of administration. Guidance values can then be developed through allocation of the TI to the various media of human exposure, based on considerations of relevant exposure profiles.

### *3.1.1 Non-threshold effects*

There is no clear consensus on appropriate methodology for the risk assessment of chemicals for which the critical effect may not have a threshold, such as genotoxic carcinogens and germ cell mutagens. A number of approaches based largely on characterization of dose response have been adopted for assessment of such effects. However, these approaches are not amenable to the development of guidance values in EHC monographs because they require socio-political judgements of acceptable health risk. Those preparing EHC and other documents for the IPCS should evaluate the relevant available data and characterize the dose-response relationship for such effects to the extent possible, based on one or more methods as considered appropriate (some approaches are described below). This should enable the development of guidance values or limits by appropriate authorities on the basis of information on such effects included in EHC monographs.

Approaches have included:

- quantitative extrapolation by mathematical modelling of the dose-response curve to estimate the risk at likely human intakes or exposures (low-dose risk extrapolation)

- relative ranking of potencies in the experimental range

- division of effect levels by an uncertainty factor.

Low-dose risk extrapolation has been accomplished by the use of mathematical models such as the Armitage-Doll multi-stage model. In more recently developed biological models, the different stages in the process of carcinogenesis have been incorporated and time to tumour has been taken into account (Moolgavkar et al., 1988). In some cases where data permit, the dose delivered to the target tissue has been incorporated into the dose-response analysis (physiologically based pharmacokinetic or PBPK modelling). It should be noted that crude expression of risk in terms of excess incidence or numbers of cancers per unit of the population at doses or concentrations much less than those on which the estimates are based may be inappropriate, owing to the uncertainties of quantitative extrapolation over several orders of magnitude. Estimated risks are believed to represent only the plausible upper bounds and vary depending upon the assumptions on which they are based.

Comparison of human exposure to the carcinogenic potency in the experimental range can also be used to indicate the magnitude of risk as a basis of derivation of guidance values. One such measure which provides a practical way to prioritize substances on the basis of their carcinogenic potency in a range close to the observed dose-response is the Exposure/Potency Index (EPI) (Health and Welfare Canada, 1992). The EPI is defined as the estimated daily human intake or exposure divided by the intake or exposure associated with a 5% incidence of tumours in experimental studies in animals or epidemiological studies in human populations (Tumorigenic $Dose_5$; $TD_5$) (Fig. 1). A calculated EPI of $10^{-6}$ represents a one million fold difference between human exposure and the intake which is at the lower end of the dose-response curve. Wherever possible, relevant toxicokinetic and mechanistic data are taken into account in the development of the EPIs.

An alternative approach is to divide the highest dose at which there is no observed increase in tumour incidence in comparison with controls by a large composite uncertainty factor (for example 5000; Weil, 1972). The magnitude of the factor could be a function of the weight of evidence (e.g., numbers of species in which the tumours have been observed or nature of the tumours). This approach is sometimes used when data on dose-response are limited.

A risk management approach which has been adopted for compounds for which the critical effect is considered not to have a threshold involves eliminating or reducing exposure as far as is practicable or to the lowest level technologically possible. Characterization of the dose-response as indicated in the procedures described above can be used in conjunction with this approach to assess the need to improve technology to reduce exposure.

### 3.1.2 *Threshold effects*

For compounds with critical effects for which there is a *threshold*, a primary objective of a review of data is to consider the comparability of experimental species and humans, and determine the highest doses or exposures that can be administered experimentally to animals or taken up by humans without producing the critical effect (see Environmental Health Criteria 70: Principles for the Safety Assessment of Food Additives and Contaminants in Food, section 5.5.1) (WHO, 1987). In studies in experimental animals, the value of the NOAEL is an observed value that is dependent on the protocol and design of the study from which it was derived. There are several "study-dependent"

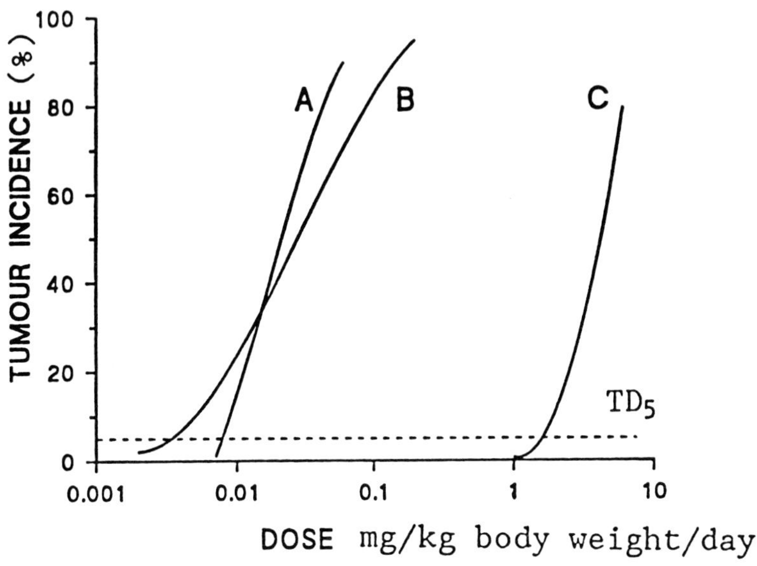


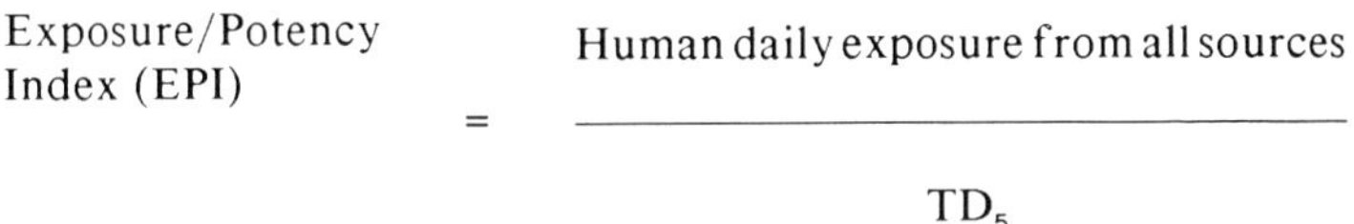

$$\text{Exposure/Potency Index (EPI)} = \frac{\text{Human daily exposure from all sources}}{TD_5}$$

Fig. 1. Dose-response curves for three hypothetical compounds showing different potencies and dose-effect relationships. The Tumorigenic Dose$_5$ ($TD_5$) provides an estimate of the dose required to produce a 5% incidence of tumours in the experimental animals.

factors that influence the magnitude of the value observed, including:

- the species, sex, age, strain and developmental status of the animals studied

- the group size
- the sensitivity of the methods used to measure the response
- the duration of exposure
- the selection of dose levels, which are frequently widely spaced, so that the observed value of the NOAEL can be in some cases considerably less than the true no-adverse-effect level.

#### 3.1.2.1 *Uncertainty factors*

There is enormous variability in the extent and nature of different data bases for risk assessment. For example, in some cases, the evaluation must be based on limited data in experimental animals; in other cases detailed information on the mechanism of toxicity and/or toxicokinetics may be available, while in some cases the risk evaluation can be based on data on effects in exposed human populations. Consequently, for the general population, the range of uncertainty factors applied in the derivation of TIs has been wide (1-10 000), although a value of 100 has been used most often. For example, the historic use of a factor of 100 based on animal studies in the absence of specific data to suggest a more appropriate value was first proposed by Lehman & Fitzhugh (1954) and later used in the derivation of ADIs for food additives by WHO (WHO, 1987; Lu, 1988). More recently, additional uncertainty factors have been incorporated to account for, for example, deficiencies in the data base, such as the absence of a NOAEL (US EPA, 1985a,b) or the absence of chronic data (NAS, 1977).

If data from well-conducted studies in human populations are the basis for the safety evaluation, a factor of 10 has been considered appropriate, as a default value (WHO, 1987). Thus the value of 100 has been regarded as comprising two factors of 10 each to allow for interspecies and inter-individual (intraspecies) variations. A scheme has been proposed which retains the two 10-fold factors as the cornerstone for extrapolating from animals to man but which allows subdivision of each to incorporate appropriate data on toxicodynamics or toxicokinetics where these exist (Renwick, 1993a) (see Fig. 2).

This approach improves the extrapolation process, and where appropriate data can be introduced, it has the effect of replacing

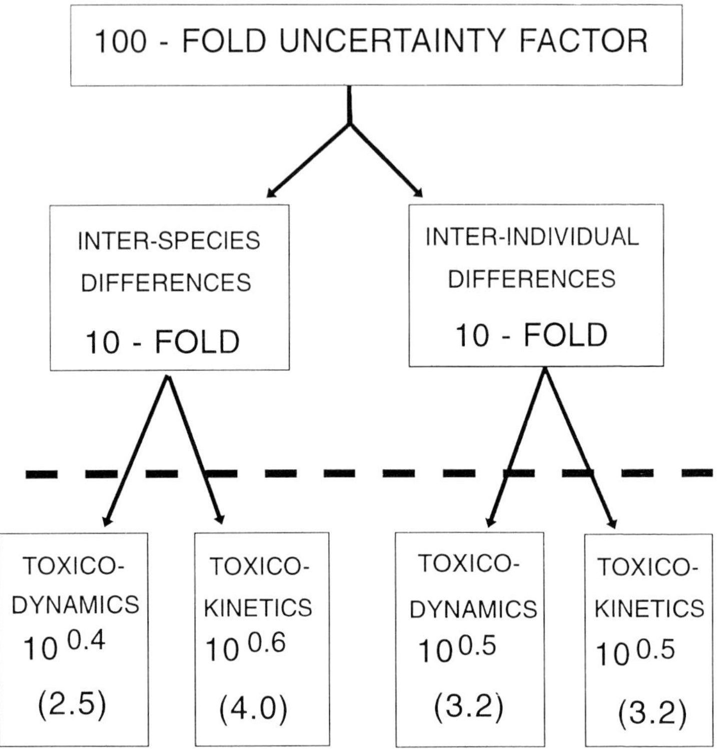


Fig. 2. Subdivision of the 100-fold uncertainty factor showing the relationship between the use of uncertainty factors (above the dashed line) and proposed subdivisions based on toxicokinetics and toxicodynamics (based on Renwick, 1993a). Actual data should be used to replace the default values if available.

"uncertainty" factors with "correction" factors. Data on differences in dynamics and kinetics between humans and common laboratory animals, such as rats, mice and dogs, indicated that there was greater potential for differences in kinetics than in dynamics so that an equal split of the 10-fold factor was inappropriate. The usual 10-fold factor (log 1) should be split into default values of 2.5 ($10^{0.4}$) for dynamics and 4 ($10^{0.6}$) for kinetics (Renwick, 1993a). A similar split was proposed for inter-individual differences between humans in toxicokinetics (pharmacokinetics) and toxicodynamics (using pharmacokinetic-pharmacodynamic modelling). However, it was considered that the variability for both aspects was similar and it was concluded that the 10-fold factor should be split evenly between both aspects, i.e. 3.2 ($10^{0.5}$) for kinetics and 3.2 ($10^{0.5}$) for dynamics. The commonly applied 100-fold uncertainty factor should be split as indicated in Fig. 2.

Precise default values for kinetics and dynamics cannot be expected on the basis of subdivision of the imprecise 10-fold composite factor. The values above are reasonable since they provide a positive value > 2 for both aspects and are compatible with the species differences in physiological parameters such as renal and hepatic blood flow. Since the data base examined was limited, it is proposed that the values for subdivision of inter-species and inter-individual variation presented in Fig. 2 be adopted on an interim basis. Adoption of the approach should encourage the development and generation of appropriate data, which could then contribute to any future revision of the default values, and further improve the scientific basis of the use of uncertainty factors.

It was recognised that appropriate toxicokinetic and toxicodynamic data are rarely available for the same compound and that to incorporate data in one area only would require the normal composite factor of 10 to be subdivided. For example, if the mechanism of action for the critical effects and differences in sensitivity between the test species and man based on *in vitro* studies were known, then these data could contribute quantitatively to the risk assessment by replacement of the default factor for interspecies differences in toxicodynamics, or differences in sensitivity (the value of 2.5 in Fig. 2) by the value indicated by the actual data. However, there could still be differences in toxicokinetics between the test species and humans so that a portion of the normal 10-fold factor would need to be retained (the value of 4 in Fig. 2).

### 1.2.2 *Relevant toxicokinetic and toxicodynamic data*

Toxicokinetics includes data on the rate and extent of absorption (bioavailability), pattern of distribution, rate and pathway of any bioactivation, and rate, route and extent of elimination. Factors such as peak plasma concentration ($C_{max}$), and area under the plasma concentration-time curve (AUC) of the toxic entity are particularly important since they are usually indicative of the extent and duration of exposure of the target organ (Renwick, 1993a). Dosimetric adjustments of administered animal dose to equivalent human dose are also possible (Jarabek et al., 1990). However it is important to define which parameter is relevant to the toxicity since some are dependent on the $C_{max}$ and not AUC (e.g., the teratogenicity of valproic acid; Nau, 1986) while for long-term bioassays, the AUC may be of greater importance. Appropriate toxicodynamic factors include the identification of the toxic entity (i.e. parent compound or a metabolite), the nature of the molecular target, the presence and activity of protective and repair mechanisms and the *in vitro* sensitivity of the target tissue (see Renwick, 1993a for details and examples). These toxicokinetic and toxicodynamic parameters should be compared between the test species and humans for derivation of interspecies factors where this is possible. Modification of the 10-fold factor for inter-individual variability in humans would require data on toxicokinetics and toxicodynamics in a wide and fully representative sample of the general or exposed population, including an assessment of neonates if appropriate.

It is emphasised that in the absence of reliable information on toxicokinetics and toxicodynamics, the default values for these factors become the commonly used composite value of 100 (i.e., 10 for inter-individual variability and 10 for interspecies variation).

#### 3.1.2.3 *Uncertainty factors for occupational exposure*

The consideration of uncertainty factors given above relates primarily to exposure of the general population. However, the general principles for derivation of TIs for occupational exposure would be somewhat similar (see, for example, Zielhuis & van der Kreek, 1979a,b; Hallenbeck & Cunningham, 1986) although they have not been widely adopted for this purpose. However, although the components of the uncertainty factor relating to the nature and severity of the toxic effect, the adequacy of the data base and interspecies variability would be similar for the development of guidance values for occupational exposure, the nature of the population exposed differs. The more vulnerable members of the human population (i.e. the very young, the sick and the elderly) do not form part of the exposed occupational population, whereas for the development of TIs for the general population, these groups must be considered. Furthermore, workplace levels and patterns of exposure can be controlled and the exposed population protected or monitored on an individual or group basis. For these reasons, it is often appropriate to use significantly lower uncertainty factors when deriving health-based limits for occupational exposure compared with those used for the development of TIs for the general population.

# 4. PROCEDURE FOR EXTRAPOLATION FROM A TOXICITY DATA BASE TO A TOLERABLE INTAKE

## 4.1 Overall procedure

The procedure, which is presented in Fig. 3, is designed to be applicable to widely differing data bases on toxicity. The procedure is also suitable for the incorporation of human data, under which circumstances some of the uncertainty factors will not be required. The scheme is presented as a series of steps, but it is important that the full data base continue to be reviewed to ensure that the final decision is appropriate. A TI for a reversible toxic effect in an animal species, for which there is complete toxicological data but without appropriate toxicokinetic or toxicodynamic data, is based on the commonly used and appropriate factor of 100. The scheme incorporates those aspects which would normally be considered in the conversion of a NOAEL (or LOAEL or equivalent) from an animal study into a TI in such a way that appropriate mechanistic or toxicokinetic data can contribute numerically to the uncertainty factor and hence to the TI.

The procedure suggested here and discussed more fully in Renwick (1993a) is based, in part, on discussions occurring over a number of years regarding the basis of uncertainty factors (see, for example, Zielhuis & van der Kreek, 1979a,b; Dourson & Stara, 1983; Lewis et al., 1990; Rubery et al., 1990). To some extent, the principles outlined here have been adopted in approaches of various national agencies (e.g., Jarabek et al., 1990; Health and Welfare Canada, 1992; US EPA, 1993).

## 4.2 Selection of pivotal study and critical effect(s)

Determination of the NOAEL, LOAEL or equivalent (possible use of benchmark dose approach) is the first step in derivation of the TI. This requires a thorough evaluation of available data on toxicity. Sophisticated detection methods may be of such sensitivity that effects can be detected at lower doses than by normal techniques; the adversity of these effects requires very careful evaluation in the determination of the NOAEL. For some chemicals, a review of the data base may reveal that two (or possibly more) adverse effects occur at low doses with NOAELs within one order of magnitude. Under such circumstances and providing: a) that the data on which the NOAELs are based are of

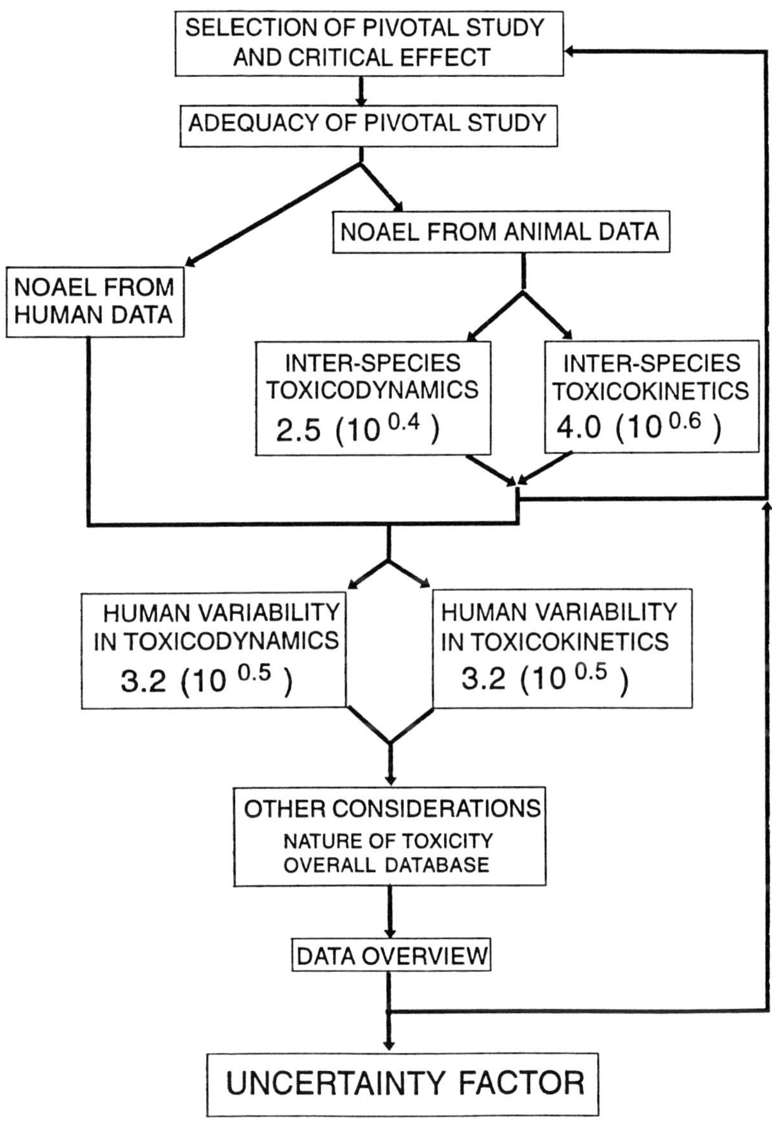


Fig. 3. Procedures for the derivation of uncertainty factors

sufficient quality to be used for risk evaluation; and b) that the NOAELs *may* require different uncertainty factors based on, for example, data on mechanisms or nature of toxicity (see below), then each effect should be considered in the following scheme and the one with the lower resulting TI used for development of guidance values. Available LOAELs within the same order of magnitude as the lowest reported NOAELs need also to be considered in this exercise since they could lead to the development of more conservative TIs.

Graphical presentation of available data can facilitate identification of effect levels relevant to development of TIs. Although the form of graphical presentation is necessarily dependent upon the size of the data base, a dose-duration graph in which NOELs, NOAELs and LOAELs are presented as a function of duration of exposure is considered to be helpful and is more fully described in Appendix 2.

## 4.3 Adequacy of the pivotal study

In situations where a NOAEL has *not* been achieved but the data on effects are of sufficient quality to be the basis of the risk assessment, then a no-adverse-effect level should be developed by the application of an appropriate uncertainty factor to the LOAEL. Uncertainty factors of 3, 5 or 10 have been used previously to extrapolate from a LOAEL to a NOAEL depending on the nature of the effect(s) and dose-response relationship (see, for example, US EPA, 1993). Alternatively, a benchmark dose may be developed by mathematical modelling of the dose-response data as an alternative to the uncertainty factor in extrapolating to the NOAEL (see Appendix 3). The pivotal study may also be considered inadequate for other reasons (e.g., duration of study, numbers of animals per group and sensitivity of the analyses of effect), and an additional uncertainty factor applied.

## 4.4 Interspecies extrapolation

In situations where appropriate toxicokinetic and/or toxicodynamic data exist for a particular compound, then the relevant uncertainty factor in Fig. 3 should be replaced by the data-derived factor. Data on PBPK and/or data on target organ exposure should be included when they are available. Subdivision of the 10-fold uncertainty factor has been used in the development of a reference concentration for 1,2-epoxybutane (US EPA, 1993). Chemicals for which the approach described here has been applied include saccharin (Renwick, 1993b), erythrosine (Poulsen, 1993), butylated hydroxyanisole (BHA) (Wurtzen, 1993) and diethylhexyl phthalate (DEHP) (Morgenroth, 1993).

If a data-derived factor is introduced then the commonly used 10-fold factor would be replaced by the product of that data-derived factor and the remaining default factor. For some classes of compounds a data-derived factor for one member of the class may be applicable to all members, thereby producing a group-based data-derived factor (see Calabrese, 1992). The interspecies uncertainty factor is not necessary if the NOAEL or LOAEL is based on human data.

## 4.5 Inter-individual variability in humans

A factor of 10 is normally used to allow for differences in sensitivity *in vivo* between the population mean and highly sensitive subjects. In cases where there are appropriate data on the inter-individual variability in toxicokinetics or toxicodynamics for a particular compound in humans, then the relevant uncertainty factor should be replaced by the data-derived factor. Data on PBPK may also be able to contribute to this assessment. If a data-derived factor is introduced, then the commonly used 10-fold factor would be replaced by the product of the data-derived factor and the remaining default factor. (For additional discussion, see Calabrese, 1985; Hattis et al., 1987).

For some compounds, it may be known that a subset of the population would be particularly sensitive, for example due to deficiencies in detoxication processes. Many of the enzymes involved in xenobiotic biotransformation are polymorphically distributed in the human population. Such polymorphism should be taken into account where the enzymatic differences result *either* in a marked change in bioavailability or clearance of the parent compound *or* in a major change in the extent of formation of the toxic entity. In cases where the default factor will not adequately cover this additional variability, then the default should be modified appropriately. Alternatively, these groups may require special strategies for health protection. In cases where the risk assessment is based on *in vivo* data in the sensitive subgroup, then the composite factor (10) should be reduced to a much lower value. A value of 1 could be used if there is an extensive data base in humans and the data base adequately addresses any identified sensitive subgroups. For example, the US EPA estimated an oral reference dose for fluoride based on the absence of dental mottling in children 12 to 14 years of age. Since this group was considered to be a sensitive subpopulation, a factor of 1 for inter-individual variation was considered to be appropriate (US EPA, 1993).

## 4.6 Other considerations

### 4.6.1 *Adequacy of the overall data base*

Major deficiencies in a toxicity data base (other than those related to the pivotal study) which increase the uncertainty of the extrapolation process should be recognized by the use of an additional uncertainty factor. Since the quality and/or completeness of different data bases vary, the additional uncertainty factor will also vary. For example, a value of 1 would be applied to a data base that was considered complete for the evaluation of the compound under consideration, but a factor of 1-100 might be necessary for limited data bases. If minor deficiencies in the data exist with respect to quality, quantity or omission, then an extra factor of 3 or 5 would be appropriate. An extra factor of 10 would be appropriate where major deficiencies in the data exist with respect to quality, quantity or omission, such as a lack of chronic toxicity studies and reproductive toxicity studies (for additional discussion see Dourson et al., 1992).

It should be appreciated that when very large uncertainty factors are incorporated, the derived TI should be considered as an very imprecise temporary estimate pending the generation of a better data base. It should be recognized that inadequacies of the pivotal study (section 4.3) could also be considered as a subset of inadequacies of the data base; the total factor for limitations of the pivotal study plus adequacy of the overall data base should not exceed 100 since such a data base is generally not acceptable for development of a TI.

### 4.6.2 *Nature of toxicity*

The nature of toxicity, i.e. whether the effect is adverse or not, is considered in the determination of NOAEL and LOAEL. For example, a concentration or dose which induces a transient increase in organ weight without accompanying biochemical or histopathological effects might be considered to be a NOAEL. If there are accompanying adverse histopathological effects in the target organ, the lowest concentration or dose at which these effects occur would be considered a LOAEL. The sensitivity of analyses of effects should also be taken into account in establishing the NOAEL or LOAEL (see discussion in section 4.2).

In addition, a number of bodies, including the WHO and FAO Joint Expert Committee on Food Additives (JECFA) and the Joint Meeting on Pesticide Residues (JMPR) have incorporated an additional "safety factor" of up to 10 (corresponding to an uncertainty factor in the current discussion) in cases where the NOAEL is derived for a critical effect which is a severe and irreversible phenomenon, such as teratogenicity or non-genotoxic carcinogenicity, especially if associated with a shallow dose-response relationship (Weil, 1972; WHO, 1987, 1990). Provision for the application of additional safety factors is included in the sequence shown in Fig. 3.

## 4.7 Final review of the total uncertainty factor

It is important that there is a final review of the total uncertainty factor applied, particularly in cases where a low value has been used, based on toxicokinetic or toxicodynamic data, to replace one of the default values. Under such circumstances, a TI derived on the basis of the appropriate overall uncertainty factor for that toxic effect might be greater than that which would be produced by an alternative, well-defined toxic end-point observed at slightly higher intakes or exposures. For this reason, there are arrows shown in Fig. 3 leading back to the data base.

## 4.8 Precision of the tolerable intake

The TI is calculated by dividing the NOAEL for the critical effect by the derived total uncertainty factor. The precision of the estimate depends in large part on the magnitude of the overall uncertainty factor used in the calculation. The precision is probably to one significant figure at best, and more usually to one order of magnitude, and for uncertainty factors of 1000 or more the precision becomes even less. Because of the imprecision of the default factors and in order to maintain credibility of the risk assessment process, the total default uncertainty factor should not exceed 10 000. If the risk assessment leads to a higher factor then the resulting TI would be so imprecise as to lack meaning. Such a situation indicates an urgent need for additional data.

## 4.9 Alternative approaches

Approaches being developed to characterize quantitatively the dose-response relationship for non-threshold effects (including the benchmark dose and categorical regression) are described in Appendix 3.

# 5. ALLOCATION OF TOLERABLE INTAKES TO DERIVE GUIDANCE VALUES

## 5.1 General considerations

Allocations of the TIs to various media for the development of guidance values are based on relative proportion of total exposure from each of the media. This necessitates the presentation of consistent and detailed estimates of exposure for as many media as possible in draft EHCs prior to review and evaluation. Wherever possible, estimation of exposure should be based on concentrations in environmental media including (but not necessarily limited to) air, food, drinking-water, soil and consumer products. With respect to soil, wherever possible, estimated exposure should take into account both ingestion and dermal contact. Since the bioavailability of contaminants in soil from both ingestion and dermal contact may be limited, this should be taken into account in assessing the contribution that soil makes to total intake from all media.

It is recommended that unless there are other age groups which are more sensitive or have widely differing exposure profiles, intake from each of the media (generally expressed as μg/kg body weight per day) should be estimated for adults, based on ICRP reference values for body weights and ingestion volumes (ICRP, 1974; Appendix 4). Wherever possible, estimation of exposure should be based on ranges of mean concentrations in environmental media on a global basis. Where data are more limited, ranges of individual values could be used. Estimates of exposure as a basis for derivation of guidance values are presented in the examples in Appendix 1.

Where the data on concentrations of a substance in environmental media are inconsistent or inadequate, exposure can be estimated based on models which incorporate as much data as possible on, for example, production, use patterns and physical and chemical properties. Models to predict distribution in environmental media and estimation of proportion of total exposure by various routes from consumer products are available (Mackay, 1991; USES, 1994). For estimation of proportions of exposure from various environmental media for development of guidance values in EHCs, it is recommended that the latest version of the Mackay level III model be used (Mackay et al., 1992). It is important that all assumptions concerning releases and physicochemical properties and limitations of the estimated proportions be clearly specified. In some cases, it may also be possible to estimate the contribution of each medium to total exposure on the basis simply of data on physical and chemical properties (e.g., for substances which are likely to be present primarily in one environmental medium).

When available, toxicokinetic data should be used to the extent possible in extrapolating across routes in the approaches to allocation described below. Dermal exposure and absorption should also be taken into account in the derivation of guidance values, although relevant data are often not available. It is also recognized that a source in one medium (e.g., potable water) may lead to additional intake from other routes (e.g., dermal and inhalation) and that, where possible, such intake should be considered in the derivation of guidance values.

In addition, total allocations of less than 100% of the TI are encouraged to account for, for example, those media for which exposure has not been characterized and cross-route exposure. The magnitude of the proportion of total intake which is not allocated should vary as a function of the adequacy of characterization of total exposure from all media.

In cases where the proportion of total exposure from a specific medium is small (less than a few percent), allocation for derivation of guidance values is not recommended since this would result in direction of risk management strategies to media which are inconsequential in contributing to total exposure.

## 5.2 General approach

The steps subsequent to development of a TI in deriving guidance values for a general population are as follows:

1. If necessary, conversion of TIs for systemic effects for different routes of exposure to a common unit for comparison based on consideration of volumes and rates of inhalation and ingestion and relevant toxicokinetic data, such as bioavailability, if available.

2. Allocation of TI to various routes and media based on estimated exposure developed on the basis of available data on measured concentrations or predicted proportions (i.e., model-derived values) to which humans are exposed. Default values can

be used in the absence of data on measured concentrations or predicted proportions of total exposure in various media.

3. Development of guidance values from intake assigned to each medium, taking into account, for instance, body weight, volume of intake and (relative) absorption efficiency (*relative* where guidance value is derived on the basis of a TI by another route of exposure). Guidance values for drinking-water are generally expressed in µg/litre or mg/litre, those in food as µg/g or mg/kg, those in air as $\mu g/m^3$ or $mg/m^3$, and those for dermal exposure as $\mu g/m^2$ surface area.

## 5.3 Detailed approach

In the following section, an approach to the allocation of tolerable intakes for development of guidance values (general population) is provided by way of example for most of the scenarios which may arise based on evaluations presented in EHCs.

The five most likely scenarios are considered to be:

### 5.3.1 Biomarkers of exposure

There is a common biomarker related to the critical effect which integrates exposure from all sources. For example, Choudhury et al. (1992) describe a model which predicts blood lead concentrations as a function of concentrations in various media.

- The contributions from the various media are determined based on a quantitative biomarker. Following allocation to various media based on an exposure scenario, guidance values are developed through incorporation of adjustment of body weight and volume of intake for each medium.

### 5.3.2 Critical effects which are not route specific

TIs have been derived for each route, e.g., TI for oral exposure ($TI_o$) and TI for inhalation ($TI_i$), and are based either on the same or on different critical effects which are not at the portal of entry. The TIs for the two routes are similar within one order of magnitude since such variation is consistent with that inherent in deriving TIs, as discussed in section 4, e.g., developmental toxicity of 2-methoxyethanol (Doe et al., 1983; Wickramaratne, 1986). This reflects the assumption that, in the absence of data to the contrary, exposure via each route is considered to contribute to a combined dose at the target site(s), i.e., additivity of dose at the target site(s).

- Allocate one TI to various media based on an exposure scenario to determine the intake in each medium on which guidance values should be based. Selection of the $TI_o$ or the $TI_i$ for this purpose should be based on either:

  a) if there is one major route of exposure then the TI for that route should be used (if there is confidence in the data base on which the exposure estimates are based); or

  b) the more conservative TI (if there is uncertainty about the relative contribution of various routes or media to total exposure).

### 5.3.3 *Difference in magnitude of effect by route of exposure*

$TI_o$ and $TI_i$ for *similar* effects vary by 1 to 2 orders of magnitude (exact magnitude of the difference for which this approach is appropriate will be dependent upon availability of additional data; e.g., manganese is more potent by inhalation than by ingestion).

- Derive the guidance values independently for each route (for example, the oral and inhalation routes, based on the $TI_o$ and $TI_i$, respectively), but allocate the proportion of the TI for each route to the appropriate medium or media based on an exposure scenario.

### 5.3.4 *Route-specific effect variation at portals of entry (due to local bioactivation or local effects)*

$TI_o$ and $TI_i$ for *route-specific* effects at the site of entry vary by 1 to 2 orders of magnitude (exact magnitude of the difference for which this approach is appropriate will be dependent upon knowledge of additional data; e.g., nasal toxicity following inhalation of acrylic acid).

- Derive the guidance values independently for each route (for example, the oral and inhalation routes, based on the $TI_o$ and $TI_i$, respectively), using the full TI for each route to the appropriate medium or media based on an exposure scenario.

### *5.3.5 Limited data base*

In this scenario, the data base is limited such that only either a $TI_o$ or a $TI_i$ can be developed.

- Allocate the available TI to various media based on an exposure scenario to determine the intake in each medium on which guidance values should be based, if the effects are qualitatively similar, if toxicokinetic data are consistent with this approach and if there are no effects at the site of entry. If any one of these criteria is not met, do not derive guidance values for the alternate route. If a TI is available for a route of exposure which does not make an important contribution to total intake, do not derive guidance values for that route.

# 6. EXAMPLES OF THE DERIVATION OF GUIDANCE VALUES

*Example 1*

The principal route of exposure is oral. Based on estimated exposure for a scenario in the general environment, 50% of total intake comes from food, 20% from water and 30% from air.

Data are adequate to establish both a $TI_o$ and a $TI_i$. The $TI_o$ and the $TI_i$ are based on similar effects and are similar (within one order of magnitude).

Allocate 50% of $TI_o$ to food to derive a guidance value for food

- multiply $TI_o$ by 0.5

Allocate 20% of $TI_o$ to water to derive a guidance value for drinking-water

- multiply $TI_o$ by 0.2

Allocate 30% of $TI_o$ to air to derive a guidance value for air

- multiply $TI_o$ by 0.3

*Example 2*

Based on an exposure scenario, 70% of total intake comes from air, 20% from water and 10% from food. The compound is also present in some consumer products but quantification of exposure is not possible. There are no data on concentrations in soil but due to its physicochemical properties, concentrations in this medium are likely to be low.

Data are sufficient to establish a $TI_i$ and a $TI_o$. The $TI_o$ and the $TI_i$ are based on similar effects and are similar to within an order of magnitude.

Convert $TI_i$ so that the values for the TIs for different routes are expressed in the same units for comparison (generally mg/kg body weight per day). This requires incorporation of information on inhalation volumes, body weight and toxicokinetic data, if available.

Use TI for principal route of exposure to derive guidance values:

Allocate 63% of $TI_i$ to air to derive a guidance value for air.

- multiply $TI_i$ by 0.63

Allocate 18% of $TI_i$ to water to derive a guidance value for drinking-water.

- multiply $TI_i$ by 0.18

Allocate 9% of $TI_i$ to food to derive a guidance value for food.

- multiply $TI_i$ by 0.09

Reserve 10% for exposure from consumer products and soil. (Wherever possible, there should be an attempt to quantitatively estimate the proportion of total intake from these sources).

Develop a guidance value for each medium by (if necessary) adjustment for body weight, volume of intake and relative absorption.

*Example 3*

The principal route of exposure is oral. Based on estimated exposure, 50% of total intake comes from food, 20% from water, 20% from air and 10% from soil (after taking bioavailability into account from the oral and dermal routes). The compound is believed not to be present in consumer products.

Data are adequate to establish both a $TI_o$ and a $TI_i$. The $TI_o$ and the $TI_i$ are based on the same effects but the compound is much more toxic by the oral route (e.g., $TI_o$ is less than the $TI_i$ by more than two orders of magnitude).

Allocate 50% of $TI_o$ to food to derive a guidance value for food

- multiply $TI_o$ by 0.5

Allocate 20% of $TI_o$ to water to derive a guidance value for drinking-water

- multiply $TI_o$ by 0.2

Allocate 10% of $TI_o$ to soil to derive a guidance value for soil

- multiply $TI_o$ by 0.1

Allocate 20% of $TI_i$ to air to derive a guidance value for air

- multiply $TI_i$ by 0.2

*Example 4*

The principal route of exposure is oral. Based on estimated exposure, 50% of total intake comes from food, 20% from water and 30% from air. There are no data indicating exposure from soil and consumer products.

Data are adequate to establish both a $TI_o$ and a $TI_i$ for route-specific effects. The $TI_o$ and the $TI_i$ are based on route-specific effects and the compound is much more toxic by the oral route (e.g., $TI_o$ is less than the $TI_i$ by more than two orders of magnitude).

Because the effects are route specific and the TIs are different by two orders of magnitude, each TI can be allocated in full to appropriate media.

Allocate 50/70 (71%) of $TI_o$ to food to derive a guidance value for food

- multiply $TI_o$ by 0.71

Allocate 20/70 (29)% of $TI_o$ to water to derive a guidance value for drinking-water

- multiply $TI_o$ by 0.29

Allocate 100% of $TI_i$ to air to derive a guidance value for air

- multiply $TI_i$ by 1

*Example 5*

The principal route of exposure is inhalation.

Data are inadequate to establish a $TI_i$.

Data are sufficient to establish a $TI_o$.

Available toxicokinetic data are inadequate for or inconsistent with extrapolation across routes.

Do not establish guidance values.

## REFERENCES


Allen BC, Van Landingham C, Howe RB, Kavlock RJ, Kimmel CA, & Faustman EM (1992) Dose-response modeling for developmental toxicity. Toxicologist, **12**(1): 300.

Allen B, Kavlock RJ, Kimmel CA, & Faustman EM (1993) Comparison of quantitative dose response modeling approaches for evaluating fetal weight changes in segment II developmental toxicity studies. Teratology, **47**(5): 41.

ATSDR (1989) Toxicological profile for aldrin/dieldrin. Atlanta, Georgia, Agency for Toxic Substances and Disease Registry (Publication ATSDR/TP-88/01).

Barnes DG & Dourson M (1988) Reference dose (RfD): Description and use in health risk assessment. Regul Toxicol Pharmacol, **8**: 471-486.

Calabrese EJ (1985) Uncertainty factors and interindividual variation. Regul Toxicol Pharmacol, **5**: 190-196.

Calabrese EJ (1992) Does the animal to human uncertainty factor incorporate interspecies differences in surface area? Regul Toxicol Pharmacol, **15**(2): 172-179.

Canada (1988) Government of Canada: Canadian Environmental Protection Act, Ottawa. Canada Gaz, II(4): 415-512.

Choudhury H, Peirano WB, Marcus A, Elias R, Griffin S, & Derosa CT (1992) Utilization of uptake biokinetic (UBK) lead model to assess risk in contaminated sites. In: Superfund risk assessment in soil contamination studies. Philadelphia, Pennsylvania, American Society of Testing and Materials, pp 193-204.

Crump KS (1984) A new method for determining allowable daily intakes. Fundam Appl Toxicol, **4**: 854-871.

Doe JE, Samuels DM, Tinston DJ, & Wickramaratne GA de S (1983) Comparative aspects of the reproductive toxicology by inhalation in rats of ethylene glycol monomethyl ether and propylene glycol monomethyl ether. Toxicol Appl Pharmacol, **69**: 43-47.

Dourson ML & Stara J (1983) Regulatory history and experimental support of uncertainty (safety) factors. Regul Toxicol Pharmacol, **3**: 224-238.

Dourson ML, Hertzberg R, Hartung R, & Blackburn K (1985) Novel methods for the estimation of acceptable daily intake. Toxicol Ind Health, **1**(4): 23-33.

Dourson ML, Knauf L, & Swartout J (1992) On reference dose (RfD) and its underlying toxicity data base. Toxicol Ind Health, **8**(3): 171-189.

Farland W & Dourson ML (1992) Noncancer health endpoints: approaches to quantitative risk assessment. In: Cothern R ed. Comparative environmental risk assessment. Boca Raton, Florida, Lewis Publishers, pp 87-106.

Gaylor DW (1989) Quantitative risk analysis for quantal reproductive and developmental effects. Environ Health Perspect, **79**: 243-246.

Gaylor DW (1992) Incidence of developmental defects at the No Observed Effect Level (NOEL). Regul Toxicol Pharmacol, **15**: 151-160.

Guth DJ, Jarabek AM, Wymer L, & Hertzberg RC (1991) Evaluation of risk assessment methods for short-term inhalation exposure. Presentation at the 84th Annual Meeting of the Air and Waste Management Association, Vancouver, British Columbia, 16-21 June 1991.

Hallenbeck WH & Cunningham KM (1986) Quantitative risk assessment for environmental and occupational health. Chelsea, Michigan, Lewis Publishers, Inc., p 199.

Hattis D, Erdreich L, & Ballew M (1987) Human variability in susceptibility to toxic chemicals - A preliminary analysis of pharmacokinetic data from normal volunteers. Risk Anal, 7(4): 415-426.

Hartung R (1986) Ranking the severity of toxic effects. In: Trace substances in environmental health. Columbia, Missouri, University of Missouri, pp 204-211.

Hartung R & Durkin PR (1986) Ranking the severity of toxic effects: Potential applications to risk assessment. Comments Toxicol, **1**: 49-63.

Health and Welfare Canada (1992) Determination of "toxic" under paragraph 11c) of the Canadian Environmental Protection Act, 1st ed. Ottawa, Ontario, Bureau of Chemical Hazards, Environmental Health Directorate.

Hertzberg RC (1989) Fitting a model to categorical response data with application to special extrapolation to toxicity. Health Phys, **57**(Suppl 1): 404-409.

Hertzberg RC & Miller M (1985) A statistical model for species extrapolation using categorical response data. Toxicol Ind Health, **1**: 43-57.

ICRP (1974) International Commission on Radiological Protection: Report of the Task Group on Reference Man. Oxford, Pergamon Press (ICRP Publication No. 23).

Jarabek AM, Menache MG, Overton JH Jr, Dourson ML, & Miller FJ (1990) The US Environmental Protection Agency's inhalation RfD methodology: Risk assessment for air toxics. Toxicol Ind Health, **6**(5): 279-301.

Kavlock RJ, Greene JA, Kimmel GL, Morrissey RE, Owens E, Rogers JM, Sadler TW, Stack F, Waters MD, & Welsch F (1991) Activity profiles of developmental toxicity: design considerations and pilot implementation. Teratology, **43**: 159-185.

Kimmel CA & Gaylor DW (1988) Issues in qualitative and quantitative risk analysis for developmental toxicology. Risk Anal, **8**: 15-20.

Lehman AJ & Fitzhugh OG (1954) 100-fold margin of safety. Assoc Food Drug Off US Q Bull, **18**: 33-35.

Lewis SC, Lynch JR, & Nikiforov AI (1990) A new approach to deriving community exposure guidelines from no-observed-adverse-effect levels. Regul Toxicol Pharmacol, **11**: 314-330.

Lu F (1988) Acceptable daily intake: inception, evolution and application. Regul Toxicol Pharmacol, **8**(1): 45-60.

Mackay D (1991) Multimedia environmental models. The fugacity approach. Chelsea, Michigan, Lewis Publishers, Inc., 260 pp.

Mackay D, Paterson S, & Shiu WY (1992) Generic models for evaluating the regional fate of chemicals. Chemosphere, **24**: 695-717.

Moolgavkar SH, Dewanji A, & Venzon DJ (1988) A stochastic two-stage model for cancer risk assessment. I: The hazard function and the probability of tumor. Risk Anal, **8**: 383-392.

Morgenroth V (1993) Scientific evaluation of the data-derived safety factors for the acceptable daily intake. Case study: diethylhexylphthalate. Food Addit Contam, **10**(3): 363-373.

NAS (1977) Drinking water and health. Washington, DC, National Research Council, US National Academy of Sciences, 939 pp.

Nau H (1986) Species differences in pharmacokinetics and drug teratogenesis. Environ Health Perspect, **70**: 113-129.

Poulsen E (1993) Case study: erythrosine. Food Addit Contam, **10**: 315-323.

Renwick AG (1993a) Data-derived safety factors for the evaluation of food additives and environmental contaminants. Food Addit Contam, **10**: 275-305.

Renwick AG (1993b) A data-derived safety (uncertainty) factor for the intense sweetener, saccharin. Food Addit Contam, **10**: 337-350.

Rubery ED, Barlow SM, & Steadman JH (1990) Criteria for setting quantitative estimates of acceptable intakes of chemicals in food in the U.K. Food Addit Contam, **7**: 287-302.

Shoaf CR (1994) US EPA inhalation testing guidelines. In: Jenkins PG, Kayser D, Muhle H, Rosner G, & Smith EM ed. Respiratory toxicology and risk assessment. Proceedings of an International Symposium. Stuttgart, Wissenschaftliche Verlagsgesellschaft mbH, pp 11-25 (IPCS Joint Series No. 18).

US EPA (1985a) National primary drinking water regulations; volatile synthetic organic chemicals; final rule and proposed rule. Fed Reg, **50**: 46830-46901.

US EPA (1985b) National primary drinking water regulations, synthetic organic chemicals, inorganic chemicals and microorganisms; proposed rule. Fed Reg, **50**: 46936-47025.

US EPA (1993) The Integrated Risk Information System (IRIS). Cincinnati, Ohio. Office of Health and Environmental Assessment, Environmental Criteria and Assessment Office.

USES (1994) Uniform system for the evaluation of substances (USES), version 1.0. Bilthoven, The Netherlands, National Institute for Public Health and Environmental Protection, 332 pp.

Waters MD, Stack HF, Brady AL, Lohman PHM, Haroun L, & Vainio H (1988) Use of computerized data listings and activity profiles of genetic and related effects in the review of 195 compounds. Mutat Res, **205**: 295-312.

Weil CS (1972) Statistics versus safety factors and scientific judgement in the evaluation for man. Toxicol Appl Pharmacol, **21**: 454-463.

WHO (1987) IPCS Environmental Health Criteria 70: Principles for the safety assessment of food additives and contaminants in food. Geneva, World Health Organization, 174 pp.

WHO (1990) IPCS Environmental Health Criteria 104: Principles for the toxicological assessment of pesticide residues in food. Geneva, World Health Organization. 117 pp.

WHO (1993) Guidelines for drinking-water quality, Second edition. Volume 1: Recommendations. Geneva, World Health Organization, 198 pp.

Wickramaratne GA de S (1986) The teratogenic potential and dose-response of dermally administered ethylene glycol monomethyl ether (EGME) estimated in rats with the Chernoff-Kavlock assay. J Appl Toxicol, **6**(3): 165-166.

Wurtzen G (1993) Scientific evaluation of the safety factor for the acceptable daily intake (ADI). Case study: butylated hydroxy anisole (BHA). Food Addit Contam, **10**: 307-314.

Zielhuis RL & van der Kreek FW (1979a) The use of a safety factor in setting health based permissible levels for occupational exposure. Int Arch Occup Environ Health, **42**: 191-201.

Zielhuis RL & van der Kreek FW (1979b) Calculation of a safety factor in setting health based permissible levels for occupational exposure. Int Arch Occup Environ Health, **42**: 203-215.

## APPENDIX 1

# EXAMPLES - DEVELOPMENT OF GUIDANCE VALUES

The following practical examples are provided to illustrate the manner in which tolerable intakes (TIs) may be developed and allocated for the derivation of guidance values for a general population (on the basis of calculated proportions of exposure from various media). In the calculation of guidance values, TIs may be rounded up to 1 or 2 significant figures depending on the quality of the data base and the extent of uncertainties involved in deriving the TI. The level of detail shown is that which is considered necessary for EHCs and should be sufficient for adaptation at national and local levels.

**Compound A**

Chlorinated hydrocarbon

*Estimates of exposure*

Estimated daily intakes of Compound A for adults (μg/kg body weight per day)[1] in the general population are as follows:

| | |
|---|---|
| Ambient air[2] | < 0.03 |
| Drinking-water[3] | 0.00007-< 0.0004 |
| Food[4] | 0.004 |
| Soil | no data |
| Consumer products | no data |
| Total Intake | 0.03 |

---

1 Assumed to weigh 64 kg, breathe 22 $m^3$ of air per day and drink 1.4 litres of water per day (ICRP, 1974) and to consume 125 g per day of a meat composite (the compound was not detected in other dietary composites).

2 Based on a mean concentration of Compound A reported in a survey of ambient air from 22 sites (< 0.10 μg/$m^3$); concentrations in indoor air were similar to those in ambient air.

3 Based on a range of mean concentrations of Compound A in drinking-water of 0.003 μg/litre to < 0.02 μg/litre.

4 Based on a concentration of 0.0018 μg/g of Compound A detected in a representative daily diet.

On the basis of these estimates, it is considered that the percentage of total exposure from various media for the general population (midpoints of estimated intakes) is as follows:

| | |
|---|---|
| outdoor/indoor air | = < 0.03/0.03 = 85.9% (86%)<br>(< 0.03 considered to be 0.03 minus intake from other media) |
| drinking-water | = 0.000245/0.03 = 0.82% (0.8%) |
| food | = 0.004/0.03 = 13.3% (13%) |
| soil | = no data |
| consumer products | = no data |

*Development of TI*

The only data identified on long-term toxicity following inhalation are the results of a single subchronic study for which no effects were observed at any concentration. Available data are considered inadequate, therefore, to establish a TI on the basis of the results of studies in which Compound A has been administered by inhalation. Moreover although the general population appears to be exposed to Compound A principally in air, based on limited available data on concentrations in food, the estimated intake in food is within the range of that estimated for air for some age groups. In addition, the principal route of intake of the most exposed age group (i.e. suckling infants) is ingestion (of mothers' milk). Owing to the lack of adequate long-term toxicity studies by the inhalation route and the possible relatively important contribution that food makes to total exposure to Compound A, a TI is derived on the basis of a long-term ingestion bioassay, as follows:

$$TI = \frac{60 \text{ mg/kg body weight per day} \times 5}{100 \times 7} \approx 0.43 \text{ mg/kg } (430\ \mu\text{g/kg}) \text{ body weight per day}$$

where:

- 60 mg/kg body weight per day is the NOAEL, determined in a well-conducted and documented long-term (chronic and carcinogenesis) bioassay, with renal tubular degeneration observed at higher doses

- 5/7 is the conversion of five days per week of dosing to seven days per week

- 100 is the uncertainty factor (×10 for inter-individual variation; ×10 for interspecies variation; available data on toxicokinetics and toxicodynamics were inadequate to modify the 10 x 10-fold uncertainty factor)

***Derivation of Guidance Values***

*Outdoor/indoor air*

The proportion of TI allocated to outdoor air based on exposure estimates = 86%

86% x TI (430 μg/kg body weight per day) = 370 μg/kg body weight per day

daily inhalation volume for adults = 22 $m^3$

mean body weight of adults = 64 kg

*Guidance value for outdoor/indoor air*

$$= \frac{370\ \mu g/kg \times 64\ kg}{22\ m^3}$$

$$= 1100\ \mu g/m^3$$

*Drinking-water*

The proportion of TI allocated to drinking-water based on exposure estimates = 0.8% (too small to permit development of meaningful guidance values since it contributes negligibly to total intake)

*Food*

The proportion of TI allocated to food based on exposure estimates = 13%

| | |
|---|---|
| 13% x TI (430 μg/kg body weight per day) | = 57 μg/kg body weight per day |

(tolerances in various foodstuffs can be developed on the basis of the amounts ingested.)

*Soil*

Owing to lack of relevant data, it is not possible to allocate a proportion of the TI to this source.

**Compound B**

Chlorinated hydrocarbon solvent

***Estimates of Exposure***

Estimated daily intakes of Compound B for adults (μg/kg body weight per day)[1] in the general population are as follows:

| | |
|---|---|
| Ambient air[2] | 0.01-0.27 |
| Indoor air[3] | 1.4 |
| Drinking-water[4] | 0.002-0.02 |
| Food[5] | 0.12 |
| Soil | no data |
| Consumer products | no data |
| Total Intake | 1.5-1.8 |

1 Assumed to weigh 64 kg, breathe 22 $m^3$ air and drink 1.4 litres of water per day (ICRP, 1974).

2 Assumed to spend 4 h/day outdoors and based on a range of mean concentrations of Compound B (0.2 to 5.0 μg/$m^3$) from a survey.

3 Assumed to spend 20 h/day indoors and based on the mean concentration of Compound B of approximately 5.1 μg/$m^3$ in the indoor air of 757 randomly selected homes examined in a survey.

4 Based on a range of mean concentrations of Compound B (0.1 to 0.9 μg/litre) in drinking-water from a number of surveys.

5 Based on the average levels of Compound B in the various composite food groups in a study on the daily intake of these food groups.

On the basis of these estimates, it is considered that the percentage of total exposure from various media for the general population (based on midpoints of estimated intakes) is as follows:

| | |
|---|---|
| outdoor air | = 0.14/1.67 = 8.3% |
| indoor air | = 1.4/1.67 = 83.8% (84%) |
| drinking-water | = 0.011/1.67 = 0.65% |
| food | = 0.12/1.67 = 7.1% |
| soil | = no data |
| consumer products | = no data |

*Development of TIs*

A Tolerable Intake for Compound B can be derived as follows:

$$TI = \frac{[(678 \text{ mg/m}^3) \times (0.043 \text{ m}^3\text{/day}) \times (6/24) \times (5/7)]}{(0.0305 \text{ kg}) \times 1000}$$

$$= 170 \ \mu\text{g/kg body weight per day}$$

where:

- 678 mg/m$^3$ is the lowest-observed-adverse-effect level (LOAEL) overall in mice determined in an adequate long-term inhalation study and based on reduced survival and hepatotoxicity in males, and lung congestion and nephrotoxicity in males and females.
- 0.043 m$^3$/day is the assumed volume of air inhaled by mice
- 6/24 and 5/7 is the conversion of 6 h/day, 5 days/week to continuous exposure.
- 0.0305 kg is the average body weight of the mice in the critical study.
- 1000 is the uncertainty factor (x10 for inter-individual variation, x10 for interspecies variation since available data on toxicokinetics and toxicodynamics were inadequate for modification of these factors, x10 for use of a LOAEL rather than a NOAEL).

In order to ensure that the TI derived on the basis of an inhalation study is sufficiently protective, another TI can be derived on the basis of studies in which Compound B was administered by ingestion. With the exception of one investigation in which reversible erythropoietic damage was reported at low concentrations (50 μg/kg body weight per day) but not confirmed in other studies, the lowest NOAEL in the longest-term (90-day) available study in which Compound B was administered orally in drinking-water to rats is 14 mg/kg body weight per day, based on effects on body weight gain, the ratio of liver or kidney weight to body weight, and serum 5′-nucleotidase activity at the next highest dose. A LOEL of 20 mg/kg body weight per day based on a slight increase in liver weight was reported in a 6-week study on mice. Values for the TI derived on the basis of the results of these two studies are within the same order of magnitude as the TI calculated from the inhalation study.

***Derivation of Guidance Values***

Since the TIs derived on the basis of studies by inhalation and ingestion are within the same range and inhalation is the most important route of exposure of the general population, the TI developed for the inhalation route will be used as the basis for derivation of guidance values.

*Outdoor air*

The proportion of TI allocated to outdoor air based on exposure estimates = 8.3%

| | |
|---|---|
| 8.3% x TI (170 μg/kg body weight per day) | = 14 μg/kg body weight per day |
| daily inhalation volume for adults | = 22 $m^3$ |
| proportion of the day spent outdoors | = 4/24 |
| volume of outdoor air inhaled daily | = 22 $m^3$ x 4/24 = 3.7 $m^3$ |
| mean body weight of adults | = 64 kg |

*Guidance value for outdoor air*

$$= \frac{14\ \mu g/kg \times 64\ kg}{3.7\ m^3}$$

$$= 242\ \mu g/m^3$$

*Indoor air*

The proportion of TI allocated to indoor air based on exposure estimates = 84%

84% x TI (170 $\mu$g/kg body weight per day) = 140 $\mu$g/kg body weight per day

daily inhalation volume for adults = 22 $m^3$

proportion of the day spent indoors = 20/24

volume of indoor air inhaled daily = 22 $m^3$ x 20/24 = 18 $m^3$

mean body weight of adults = 64 kg

*Guidance value for indoor air*

$$= \frac{140\ \mu g/kg \times 64\ kg}{18\ m^3}$$

$$= 498\ \mu g/m^3$$

*Drinking-water*

The proportion of TI allocated to drinking-water based on exposure estimates = 0.65% (too small to permit development of meaningful guidance values since it contributes negligibly to total intake)

*Food*

The proportion of TI allocated to food based on exposure estimates = 7.1%

7.1% x TI (170 μg/kg body weight per day) = 12 μg/kg body weight per day or 10 μg/kg body weight per day to one significant figure

(tolerances in various foodstuffs could then be developed on the basis of amounts ingested.)

*Soil*

Owing to lack of relevant data, it is not possible to allocate a proportion of the TI to this source.

**Compound C**

Naturally occurring inorganic chemical

***Estimates of Exposure***

The percentage of total exposure from various media for adults in the general population in country 1 is as follows:

| | |
|---|---|
| outdoor/indoor air | = 0.02% |
| drinking-water | = 6.9% |
| food | = 80% |
| soil | = 0.11% |
| consumer products | = 12.8% |

In contrast, the percentage of total exposure from various media for adults in the general population in one area in country 2 is as follows:

| | |
|---|---|
| outdoor/indoor air | = 35% |
| drinking-water | = 11% |
| food | = 55% |

***Development of TIs***

It is concluded, on the basis of data from several studies in human populations, that the TI is 200 μg/kg body weight per day.

***Derivation of Guidance Values - Country 1***

*Outdoor/indoor air*

The proportion of TI allocated to air based on exposure estimates = 0.02% (too small to permit development of meaningful guidance values)

*Drinking-water*

The proportion of TI allocated to drinking-water based on exposure estimates = 6.9%

| | |
|---|---|
| 6.9% x TI (200 μg/kg body weight per day) | = 13.8 μg/kg body weight per day |
| daily volume of ingestion of drinking-water for adults in Country 1 | = 1.5 litres |
| mean body weight of adults in Country 1 | = 70 kg |

*Guidance value for drinking-water*

$$= \frac{13.8\ \mu g/kg \times 70\ kg}{1.5}$$

$$= 644\ \mu g/litre$$

*Food*

The proportion of TI allocated to food based on exposure estimates = 80%

| | |
|---|---|
| 80% x TI (200 μg/kg body weight per day) | = 160 μg/kg body weight per day or 200 μg/kg body weight per day to one significant figure |

(tolerances in various foodstuffs can then be developed on the basis of amounts ingested.)

*Soil*

The proportion of TI allocated to air based on exposure estimates = 0.11%

(too small to permit development of meaningful guidance values)

*Consumer products*

The proportion of TI allocated to consumer products based on exposure estimates = 12.8%

| | |
|---|---|
| 12.8% x TI (200 μg/kg body weight per day) | = 26 μg/kg body weight per day |

(limits in consumer products can be developed on the basis of patterns of use.)

***Derivation of Guidance Values - Country 2***

*Outdoor/indoor air*

The proportion of TI allocated to air based on exposure estimates = 35%

| | |
|---|---|
| 35% x TI (200 μg/kg body weight per day) | = 70 μg/kg body weight per day |
| daily inhalation volume for adults in Country 2 | = 20 $m^3$ |
| mean body weight of adults in Country 2 | = 60 kg |

*Guidance value for outdoor/indoor air*

$$= \frac{70\ \mu g/kg \times 60\ kg}{20\ m^3}$$

$$= 210\ \mu g/m^3$$

*Drinking-water*

The proportion of TI allocated to drinking-water based on exposure estimates = 11%

| | |
|---|---|
| 11% x TI (200 μg/kg body weight per day) | = 22 μg/kg body weight per day |

daily volume of ingestion of drinking-water for adults in Country 2 = 1.5 litres

mean body weight of adults in Country 2 = 60 kg

*Guidance value for drinking-water*

$$= \frac{22\ \mu g/kg \times 60\ kg}{1.5}$$

= 880 μg/litre

*Food*

The proportion of TI allocated to food based on exposure estimates = 55%

55% x TI (200 μg/kg body weight per day) = 110 μg/kg body weight per day

(tolerances in various foodstuffs can be developed on the basis of amounts ingested.)

*Soil*

No data are available.

*Consumer products*

No data are available.

APPENDIX 2

# GRAPHICAL APPROACHES

The use of graphs of dose-effect and dose-response toxicity data to complement the text discussion in the development of TIs and guidance values is considered valuable. Such graphs can display an overview of the full range of dose-response information. Graphs can range from simple "thermometer" presentations as employed by the US Agency for Toxic Substances and Disease Registry (ATSDR, 1989), to dose-effect and dose-response graphs for specific toxic effects such as genotoxicity (Waters et al., 1988) or developmental toxicity (Kavlock et al., 1991), or to dose-duration graphs described by Hartung (1986), Hartung & Durkin (1986), and Dourson et al. (1985).

Fig. 4 is an example of a dose-duration graph and presents data for methoxychlor adapted from Dourson et al. (1985). This figure summarizes the available frank-effect levels (FEL), adverse-effect levels (AEL), no-observed-adverse-effect levels (NOAEL), and no-observed-effect levels (NOEL). Adverse-effect levels are presented as a function of both dose in mg/day and exposure as a fraction of lifespan.

Each point in the graph represents one dose group from one study. The size of the point is a rough indication of its usefulness for determining tolerable intakes, where larger points indicate more useful information. Other information includes target organs. These data can also be used to estimate a best fitting line for NOAEL across duration.

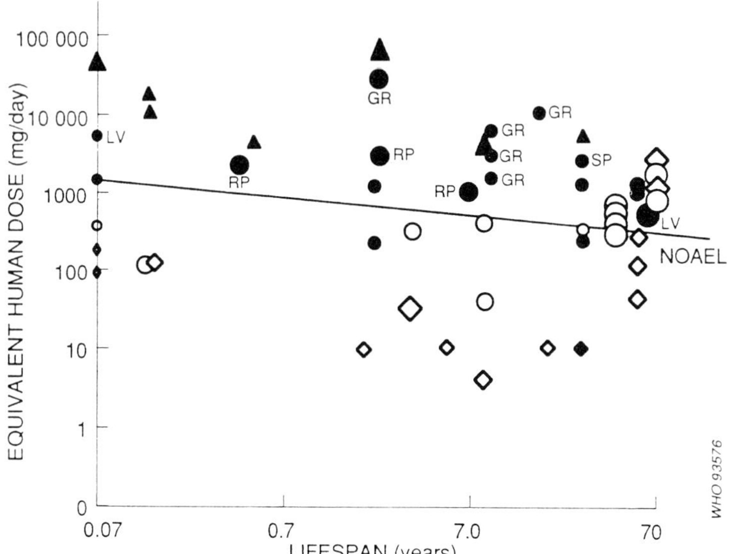


Fig. 4. Effect-dose-duration plot of all relevant human and animal oral toxicity data for methoxychlor. Effect levels are shown for different targets (LV = liver, RP = reproductive organ, GR = growth reduction, SP = spleen). Animal doses have been converted by a body surface area factor to approximate the equivalent human dose. Dose durations are divided by the appropriate species lifespan to yield a fraction which, when multiplied by 70 years (the assumed average human lifespan), gives the corresponding position on the *x* axis, i.e. a lifetime exposure study in any species would be shown as 70 years. Study usefulness is denoted by symbol size. Effect levels, listed in order of decreasing severity, are:

- ▲ Frank-effect level (FEL)
- ● Adverse-effect level (AEL)
- O No-observed-adverse-effect level (NOAEL)
- ◇ No-observed-effect level (NOEL)

(based on Dourson et al., 1985)

**APPENDIX 3**

# ALTERNATIVE APPROACHES

Alternative approaches being considered in the derivation of TIs for threshold effects include the benchmark dose and categorical regression.

## Benchmark dose

The benchmark dose (BD) is the lower confidence limit (LCL) of the dose that produces a small increase in the level of adverse effects (e.g., 5 or 10%; Crump, 1984) to which uncertainty factors (UF) can be applied to develop a tolerable intake (see Fig. 5, adapted from Kimmel & Gaylor, 1988).

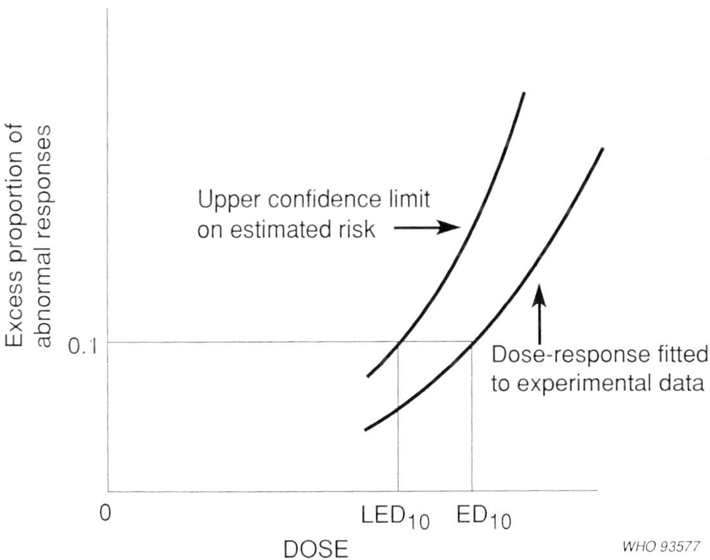


Fig. 5. Graphical illustration of benchmark dose (BD). In this example $LED_{10}$ = BD. BD could also be calculated as $LED_{05}$, $LED_{01}$ or other values. ED stands for effective dose. (Adapted from Kimmel & Gaylor, 1988)

The BD has a number of advantages over the NOAEL. Firstly, it is derived on the basis of data from the entire dose-response curve for the critical effect rather than that from the single dose group at the NOAEL (i.e. one of the few (usually three) preselected dose levels). Use of the BD also facilitates comparison of studies on the same agent or the potencies of different agents. The BD can also be calculated from data sets in which a NOAEL was not determined, eliminating the need for an additional uncertainty factor to be applied to the LOAEL. Lastly, definition of the BD as a lower confidence limit accounts for the statistical power and quality of the data. That is, the confidence intervals around the dose-response curve for studies with small numbers of animals and, therefore, lower statistical power would be wide; similarly, confidence intervals in studies of poor quality with highly variable responses would also be wide. In either case, the wider confidence interval would lead to a lower BD, reflecting the greater uncertainty of the data base. On the other hand, narrow confidence limits (reflecting better studies) would result in higher BDs.

One of the chief disadvantages of this approach is that it is not possible to determine a BD for many types of data on toxicity (e.g., histopathological data).

Several methods have been published for determining both the dose-response curve from which the BD is derived and appropriate uncertainty factors to estimate the TI (e.g., Crump, 1984; Dourson et al., 1985; Kimmel & Gaylor, 1988; Gaylor, 1989; Allen et al., 1992). However, there is as yet, no consensus on the incidence of effect to be used as a basis for the BD, although it should be comparable to the level of effect typically associated with the NOAEL. For data bases on developmental toxicity, it has been estimated that this level of effect is in the range of 1-10% (Crump, 1984; Gaylor, 1989, 1992); this range is similar for other toxic end-points (Farland & Dourson, 1992; Shoaf, 1994). Allen et al. (1992, 1993) have estimated that a BD calculated from the LCL at 5% is, on average, comparable to the NOAEL, whereas choosing a BD from the LCL at 10% is more representative of a LOAEL (Farland & Dourson, 1992). Choosing a BD that is comparable to the NOAEL has two advantages: (i) it is within the experimental dose-range, eliminating the need to interpolate the dose-response curve to low levels; and (ii) justification of the application of similar UFs as are currently applied to the NOAEL for interspecies and inter-individual variation.

**Categorical Regression**

The theory and application of categorical regression has been addressed by Hertzberg & Miller (1985), Hertzberg, (1989), Guth et al. (1991) (inhalation exposure to methylisocyanate), and Farland & Dourson (1992) (oral exposure to arsenic). Data on toxicity are classified into one of several categories, such as NOEL, NOAEL, AEL or FEL, or others, as appropriate. These categories are then regressed on the basis of dose and, if required, duration of exposure. The result is a graph of probability of a given category of effect with dose or concentration, which is useful in the analysis of potential risks above the TI, especially for comparisons amongst chemicals.

Depending on the extent of the available data on toxicity, additional estimations regarding the percentage of individuals with specific adverse effects are possible. Such estimations require, however, an understanding of the mechanisms of toxicity of the critical effect, knowledge of the extrapolation between the experimental animal and man, and/or incidences of specific effects in humans.

Similar to the BD, categorical regression utilizes information from the entire dose-response curve, resulting in more precise estimates of risk when compared to the current approach (NOAEL-based TIs). However, categorical regression requires more information than the current TI method, and the interpretation of the probability scale can be problematic.

APPENDIX 4

# BODY WEIGHT AND VOLUMES OF INTAKE FOR REFERENCE MAN

*(based on ICRP, 1974, unless otherwise indicated)*

**Body weight, kg**

| | |
|---|---|
| Adult male | = 70 |
| Adult female | = 58 |
| Average | = 64[a] |

**Daily fluid intake (milk, tap water, other beverages), ml/day**

*Normal conditions*:

| | |
|---|---|
| Adults | = 1000-2400, representative figure = 1900[b] (excluding milk: 1400[c]) |
| Adult male | = 1950 |
| Adult female | = 1400 |
| Child (10 years) | = 1400 |

*High average temperature (32 °C)*:

| | |
|---|---|
| Adults | = 2840-3410 |

*Moderate activity*:

| | |
|---|---|
| Adults | = 3700 |

**Respiratory volumes**

*8-h respiratory volume, litres*

| | | |
|---|---|---|
| resting: | Adult man | = 3600 |
| | Adult woman | = 2900 |
| | Child (10 years) | = 2300 |
| light/non-occupational activity: | Adult man | = 9600 |
| | Adult woman | = 9100 |
| | Child (10 years) | = 6240 |

*Daily inhalation volume, $m^3$*

(8-h resting, 16-h light/non-occupational activity)

| | |
|---|---|
| Adult male | = 23 |
| Adult female | = 21 |
| Child (10 years) | = 15 |
| Average adult | = 22 |

Proportion of time spent indoors[c] = 20 h/day

**Amount of soil ingested**[c] = 20 mg/day

**Dietary intake**[d]

| | |
|---|---|
| Cereals | = 323 g/day (flour and milled rice) |
| Starchy roots | = 225 g/day (sweet potatoes, cassava and other) |
| Sugar | = 72 g/day (includes raw sugar, excludes syrups and honey) |
| Pulses and nuts | = 33 g/day (includes cocoa beans) |
| Vegetables and fruits | = 325 g/day (fresh equivalent) |
| Meat | = 125 g/day (includes offal, poultry and game in terms of carcass weight, excluding slaughter fats) |
| Eggs | = 19 g/day (fresh equivalent) |
| Fish | = 23 g/day (landed weight) |
| Milk | = 360 g/day (excludes butter; includes milk products as fresh milk equivalent) |
| Fats and oils | = 31 g/day (pure fat content) |

[a] WHO uses 60 kg for calculation of acceptable daily intakes and water quality guidelines (WHO, 1987, 1993).

[b] WHO uses a daily per capita drinking-water consumption of 2 litres in calculating water quality guidelines (WHO, 1993)

[c] From Health and Welfare Canada (1992)

[d] Based on average of estimates for 7 geographical regions (ICRP, 1974)

# RESUME

Des valeurs guides devraient être établies dans les Critères d'hygiène de l'environnement (CHE) de l'IPCS pour l'exposition aux produits chimiques présents dans l'environnement. Ces valeurs guides pourront être modifiées par les autorités nationales et locales lorsque celles-ci fixeront leurs normes et limites pour les différents milieux. L'élaboration des valeurs guides pour les produits chimiques comporte les étapes suivantes:

1. Evaluer et résumer les données relatives à la toxicité pour l'homme et l'animal et à l'exposition humaine qui offrent un intérêt particulier pour le calcul des valeurs guides. Ces données devraient de préférence être présentées sous la forme d'un texte explicatif résumant les points cruciaux, complété par des graphiques.

2. Ces données pourront servir à calculer une dose tolérable (DT) pour les différentes voies d'exposition dans le cas des effets pour lesquels on considère qu'il existe un seuil. Le calcul consiste généralement à appliquer des facteurs d'incertitude aux doses sans effet indésirable observé (DSEIO) établies par l'étude la plus pertinente pour les effets critiques. En ce qui concerne les effets pour lesquels il n'existe pas de seuil, la relation dose-réponse devra être caractérisée aussi complètement que possible.

3. Estimer la proportion de la dose totale provenant des différents milieux (atmosphère à l'intérieur des locaux, air ambiant, nourriture, eau, etc.) dans une situation donnée, en prenant comme base de calcul un ensemble cohérent de données sur les volumes théoriques absorbés par l'"homme de référence" de la Commission internationale de protection contre les radiations (CIPR) et des concentrations représentatives de l'environnement général. En l'absence de données adéquates sur les concentrations dans les différents milieux, on pourra utiliser des modèles mathématiques pour estimer la répartition entre ces milieux.

4. Attribuer une proportion de la DT aux différents milieux (d'après les résultats de l'estimation décrite à l'étape 3 ci-dessus) de façon à déterminer la dose ou l'exposition attribuable à chaque milieu.

5. Etablir des valeurs guides pour les doses attribuées à chaque milieu en tenant compte éventuellement du poids corporel, du volume absorbé et de l'efficacité de l'absorption (efficacité

d'absorption *relative* lorsque la valeur guide est calculée à partir de la DT établie pour une autre voie d'exposition). Dans les monographies de la série CHE, les valeurs guides devraient être établies pour un scénario d'exposition clairement défini, fondé sur les données applicables à l'homme de référence de la CIPR, données qui ne sont pas nécessairement représentatives des conditions nationales ou locales d'exposition. Normalement, les valeurs guides seront calculées pour une population générale représentative, soumise à des conditions d'exposition également représentatives. Elles devront être adaptées au niveau national et local en fonction des circonstances.

6. La base de calcul des DT et des valeurs guides devrait être clairement expliquée dans les monographies de la série CHE (pour le niveau de détail exigé, voir les exemples de l'appendice 1).

# RESUMEN

En los monografías de la serie Criterios de Salud Ambiental (EHC) del IPCS deben formularse valores orientativos para la exposición a sustancias químicas presentes en el medio ambiente, valores que las autoridades nacionales y locales pueden modificar al determinar sus límites y normas aplicables al medio. Los pasos previstos para cualquier sustancia química son los siguientes:

1. Evaluar y resumir la información referente a la toxicidad en los animales y el hombre y la exposición en el hombre, seleccionando la más pertinente para el cálculo de los valores orientativos. El esquema más apropiado para presentar los datos pertinentes con miras al cálculo de los valores orientativos es un texto que describa sucintamente los datos críticos, complementado con los gráficos oportunos.

2. Calcular a partir de esos datos una Ingesta Tolerable (IT) para las diversas vías de exposición y para los distintos efectos que se considere que tienen un umbral. Ello entraña el uso de factores de incertidumbre, aplicados por lo general al nivel sin efectos adversos observados (NOAEL) para los efectos críticos referidos en el estudio más pertinente. En el caso de los efectos sin umbral, se caracterizará en la medida de lo posible la relación dosis-respuesta.

3. Estimar la proporción de ingesta total que tiene su origen en los diversos medios (p. ej., aire de espacios interiores y ambiental, alimentos y agua), sobre la base de las exposiciones calculadas para un conjunto coherente de volúmenes supuestos de ingesta (utilizando el hombre de referencia de la Comisión Internacional de Protección contra las Radiaciones (CIPR)) y de concentraciones representativas en el medio ambiente general para una determinada situación. Si no se dispone de datos suficientes sobre las concentraciones en diversos medios, pueden emplearse modelos matemáticos para estimar la distribución por esos medios.

4. Asignar una proporción de la IT a diversos medios de exposición (basándose en la exposición estimada conforme a lo explicado en el paso 3 precedente) para determinar la ingesta o exposición en cada medio.

5. Formular valores orientativos a partir de las ingestas asignadas a cada medio, teniendo en cuenta (si es necesario) el peso corporal, el volumen de ingesta y la eficiencia de absorción (la eficiencia de

absorción *relativa* cuando para calcular el valor orientativo se utilice la IT correspondiente a otra vía de exposición). En los monografías de la serie EHC se formularían valores orientativos para unas condiciones de exposición claramente definidas, basadas en los datos del hombre de referencia de la CIPR y no necesariamente representativas de las condiciones de exposición nacionales o locales. Se calcularán comúnmente valores orientativos para una población general representativa y unas condiciones de exposición representativas. Los valores orientativos se deberán adaptar a nivel nacional y local según proceda en función de las circunstancias locales.

6. En los monografías de la serie EHC se deberán detallar claramente los fundamentos del cálculo tanto de la IT como de los valores orientativos (respecto al grado de detalle, véanse los ejemplos presentados en el apéndice 1).